Mediterranean Lunch Cookbook

A collection of 50 delicious recipes for your Mediterranean Diet

Carlo Montesanti

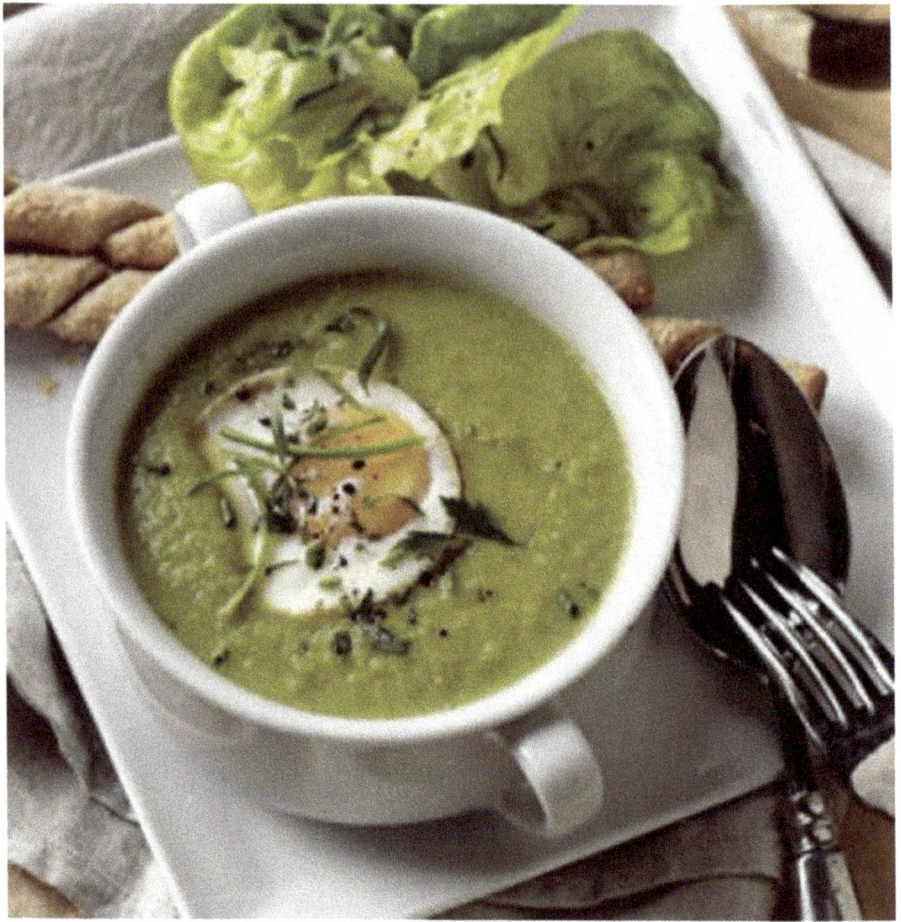

Table of Contents

Spring soup with a poached egg

Prep Time: 20 min

Cook Time: 20 min

Serve: 6

Ingredients:

- 3 tbsp Olive Oil

- 2 Leeks

- 6 Eggs

- 2 tbsp splash Vinegar

- 3 Carrots

- 6 cups Chicken Stock

- One bunch Asparagus

- One bunch Ramps root

- 2 Garlic cloves

- 1/2 Sugar Snap Peas

- 1/2 Mixed Herbs Lemon Juice

Preparation:

1. Heat olive oil in a soup pot, then add carrots, leeks, garlic, and the diced ramp stalks. Flavor with salt & cook on over -high temp. Unless it softens, & the garlic starts to turn golden about 5 minutes. Add the stock and bring to a boil, then reduce to a simmer. Simmer until the vegetables are tender, about 10 minutes.

2. Add the asparagus & pea pods & continue to simmer until the asparagus & peas are crisp-tender, about three mints.

3. Add a pinch of salt & a splash of vinegar. Crack an egg into a cup & gently lower into the simmering water. Turn off the heat, cover the frypan, & let the eggs poach for 4 minutes.

4. Remove eggs & place one egg in the bottom of every soup bowl. Finally, remove from stove & mix the ramp herbs & leaves. Taste & season as needed with sea salt, pepper, & lemon juice. Serve & enjoy your soup.

Mint avocado chilled soup

Prep Time: 5 min

Cook Time: 0 min

Serve: 2

Ingredients:

- 1 cup of milk chilled

- 1 tbsp lime juice

- 20 mint leaves

- One ripe avocado

- Two romaine lettuce leaves

- Salt to taste

Preparation:

Put all ingredients in blender & mix them well. The soup should be dense but not as dense as a puree. Freeze in the fridge for five to ten minutes & serve it.

Cucumber olive rice

Prep Time: 30 min

Cook Time: 55 min

Serve: 8

Ingredients:

- Three garlic cloves

- 1 lb. heirloom

- 8 oz feta

- 1 cup parsley leaves

- 7 tbsp olive oil

- Kosher salt to taste

- Black pepper to taste

- 1.5 cups brown rice

- One chopped onion

- Three chopped cucumbers

- 3 tbsp sherry vinegar

- 1 cup mint leaves

Preparation:

1. Add 2 tbsp. Oil in a heated frying pan. Then add garlic along with salt and cook it for five minutes. While stirring till it gives aroma & transparent. Transfer this into a bowl

2. Take frying pan again, heat it and add 1 tbsp of oil & rice. Cook this for three minutes while stirring till it turns golden & nutty.

3. Add water to the bowl and boil it. Mix it only one time & then decrease the heat to low temp. and then cover it. Cook till rice is delicate, & water has been soaked up. Please remove it from the stove and let it cool for five minutes.

4. Move rice into a bowl along with the mixture of onion and let it cool for 20 minutes.

5. Mix cucumbers, tomatoes, vinegar, & remaining oil. Season with sea salt & black pepper. Finally, Coat with cheese, parsley, & mint and serve it.

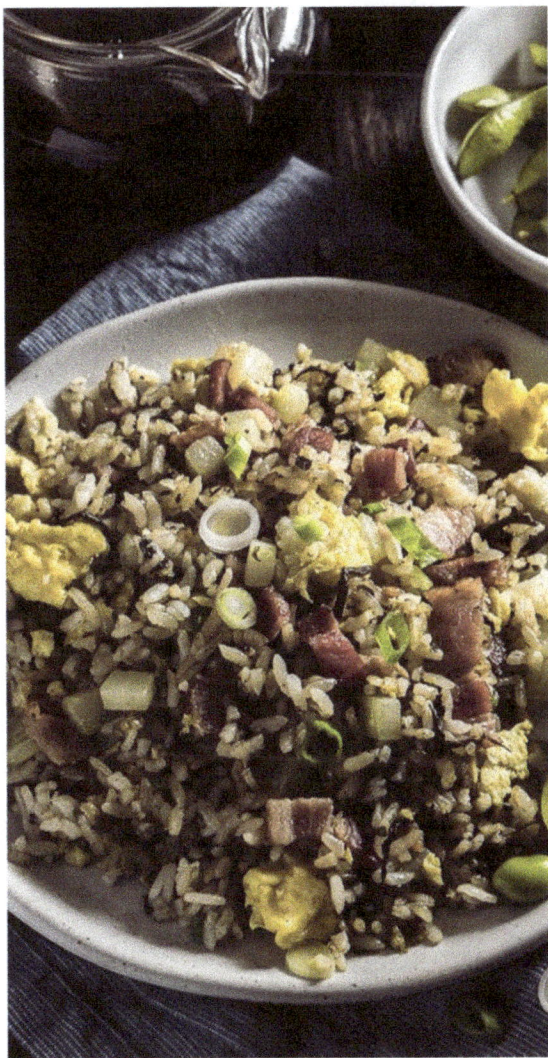

Basil tomato rice

Prep Time: 10 min

Cook Time: 30 min

Serve: 4

Ingredients:

- 1 tbsp olive oil

- Two cloves garlic salt to taste

- Black pepper to taste

- 1/2 cup onion

- 1 cup white rice

- One ripe tomato

- 2 cups chicken broth

- 3 tbsp grated parmesan cheese

- 2 tbsp basil

Preparation:

1. Take a frying pan, add onions & olive oil to it and cook it for four minutes. Then add rice in it & cook it for 2-3 mints more. Add tomatoes, chicken broth, sale, black pepper & garlic to it.

2. Cover it and boil & reduce heat to a simmer. Cook for 20 minutes. Without raising the lid. Please remove it from the stove & rest it for five minutes before removing the lid off. Add parmesan cheese & basil & mix well.

3. Place this in a bowl and garnish it with remaining parmesan cheese along with basil & tomatoes if required.

Watermelon Bowl

Prep Time: 1 h 10 min

Cook Time: 0 min

Serve: 32

Ingredients:

- 1 Watermelon, Halved Lengthwise

- 3 Tablespoons Lime Juice, Fresh

- 1 Cup Sugar

- 1 ½ Cup Water

- 1 ½ Cups Mint Leaves, Fresh & Chopped

- 6 Plums, Pitted & Halved

- 1 Cantaloupe, Small

- 4 Nectarines, Pitted & Halved

- 1 lb. Green Grapes, Seedless

Preparation:

1. Mix sugar and water in a two-quart pot and bring it to a boil using medium heat. Stir your sugar in until it dissolves. Mix in your lime juice and mint, and then place it in the fridge until chilled. Chop your watermelon and cantaloupe into bite sized pieces, and then slice the nectarines and plums into wedges.

2. Mix all your fruit in a large bowl before adding in your grapes. Take the mixture out of the fridge and pour it over the fruit. Mix well, and then cover it with saran wrap.

3. Refrigerate for two hours, and stir occasionally. Serve chilled.

Red Egg Skillet

Prep Time: 5 min

Cook Time: 10 min

Serve: 6

Ingredients:

- 7 Greek Olives, Pitted & Sliced

- 3 Tomatoes, Ripe & Diced

- 2 Tablespoons Olive oil

- 4 Eggs

- ¼ Cup Parsley, Fresh & Chopped

- 1/8 Teaspoon Sea Salt

- Fine Black Pepper to Taste

Preparation:

1. Get out a pan and grease it. Throw your tomatoes in and cook for ten minutes before adding in your olives. Cook for another five minutes.

2. Add your eggs into the pan, cooking over medium-heat so that your eggs are cooked all the way through.

Season with salt and pepper and serve topped with parsley.

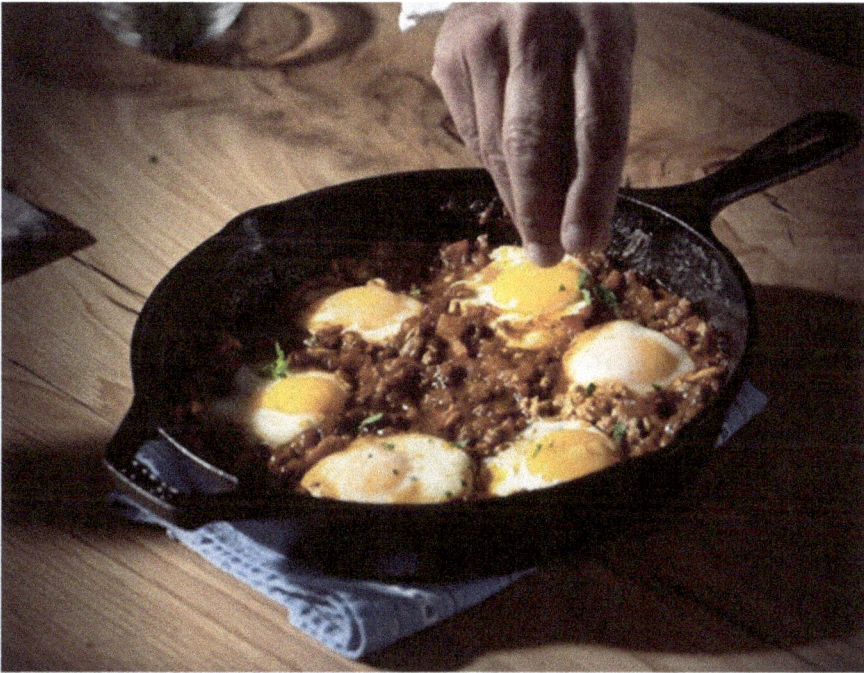

Grecian "Golden Delicious"

Dessert

Prep Time: 10 min

Cook Time: 35 min

Serve: 8

Ingredients:

- 1½-lbs. Golden Delicious apples, peeled, cored, and sliced thinly (divided)

- pcs eggs

- Zest of lemon, grated

- ⅓ -cup brown sugar

- A pinch of salt

- ¼-cup plus 1-tbsp low-fat milk

- 3-tsp baking powder

- 1 cup less

- 1-tbsp whole-wheat flour, sifted

- 1-tbsp light brown sugar for topping (optional)

- 1-tbsp icing sugar for dusting

Preparation:

1. Preheat your oven to 350 °F. Prepare a greased and flour-sprinkled 8" x 8" baking pan. Set aside. Combine and mix the eggs, lemon zest, sugar, and salt in your stand mixer's mixing bowl. Beat to a creamy and thick consistency.

2. Pour in the milk, and add the baking powder and flour. Beat until fully incorporated. Add ⅔ or 1-pound of the sliced apples to the batter. By using a spatula, mix thoroughly until fully combined. Transfer the batter in the prepared baking pan. Top the batter with the remaining apple slices. If desired, sprinkle with a tablespoon of brown sugar.

3. Place the pan in the preheated oven. Bake for 35 minutes until an inserted toothpick into the center of the apple cake

comes out clean. To serve, dust the low-fat cake with icing sugar.

Chocolate Covered Strawberries

Prep Time: 15 min

Serve: 24 servings

Ingredients:

- 16 ounces milk chocolate chips
- 2 tablespoons shortening
- 1-pound fresh strawberries with leaves

Preparation:

1. In a bain-marie, melt chocolate and shorter, occasionally stirring until smooth. Hold them by the toothpicks and immerse the strawberries in the chocolate mixture.

2. Put toothpicks in the top of the strawberries.

3. Turn the strawberries and put the toothpick in the styrofoam so that the chocolate cools.

Strawberry Angel Food Dessert

Prep Time: 15 min

Serve: 18

Ingredients:

- 1 angel cake (10 inches)

- 2 packages of softened cream cheese

- 1 cup of white sugar

- 1 container (8 oz) of frozen fluff, thawed

- 1 liter of fresh strawberries, sliced

- 1 jar of strawberry icing

Preparation:

1. Crumble the cake in a 9 x 13-inch dish.

2. Beat the cream cheese and sugar in a medium bowl until

the mixture is light and fluffy. Stir in the whipped topping.

3. Crush the cake with your hands, and spread the cream cheese mixture over the cake.

4. Combine the strawberries and the frosting in a bowl until the strawberries are well covered. Spread over the layer of cream cheese. Cool until ready to serve.

Fruit Pizza

Prep Time: 30 min

Serve: 8

Ingredients:

- Sugar cookie dough in a cooled package of 1 oz (18 oz)

- cream cheese in a package of 1 (8 ounces), softened

- 1 (8 oz.) Frozen defrosted filling, defrosted

- 2 cups of freshly cut strawberries

- 1/2 cup of white sugar

- 1 pinch of salt

- 1 tablespoon corn flour

- 2 tablespoons lemon juice

- 1/2 cup orange juice

- 1/4 cup water

- 1/2 teaspoon orange zest

Preparation:

1. Preheat the oven to 175 ° C (350 ° F). Slice the cookie dough then place it on a greased pizza pan. Press the dough flat into the mold. Bake for 10 to 12 minutes. Let cool.

2. Soften the cream cheese in a large bowl and then stir in the whipped topping. Spread over the cooled crust. You can relax for a moment at this stage or continue to arrange the fruit. Start with strawberries cut in half. Place them in a circle around the outer edge. Continue with the fruit of your choice by going to the center. If you use bananas, immerse them in lemon juice so that they do not get dark. Then make a sauce with a spoon on the fruit.

3. Combine sugar, salt, corn flour, orange juice, lemon juice, and water in a pan. Boil and stir over medium heat. Bring to the boil and cook for 1 or 2 minutes until thick.

Remove from heat and add the grated orange zest. Cool, but not in place. Place on the fruit.

4. Allow to cool for two hours, cut into quarters, and serve.

Bananas Foster

Prep Time: 5 min

Serve: 4

Ingredients:

- 2/3 cup dark brown sugar

- 1/4 cup butter

- 3 1/2 tablespoons rum

- 1 1/2 teaspoon vanilla extract

- 1/2 teaspoon of ground cinnamon

- 3 bananas, peeled and cut lengthwise and broad

- 1/4 cup coarsely chopped nuts1, vanilla ice cream

Preparation:

1. Melt the butter in a big, deep frying pan over medium heat. Stir in sugar, rum, vanilla, and cinnamon.

2. When the mixture starts to bubble, place the bananas and nuts in the pan. Bake until the bananas are hot, 1 to 2 minutes. Serve immediately on a vanilla ice cream.

Cranberry Orange Cookies

Prep Time: 20 min

Serve: 48

Ingredients:

- 1 cup of soft butter
- 1 cup of white sugar
- 1/2 cup brown sugar
- 1 egg
- 1 teaspoon grated orange peel
- 2 tablespoons orange juice
- 2 1/2 cups flour
- 1/2 teaspoon baking powder
- 1/2 teaspoon salt
- 2 cups chopped cranberries
- 1/2 cup chopped walnuts (optional)

- 1/2 teaspoon grated orange peel

- 3 tablespoons orange juice

- 1 ½ cup confectioner's sugar

Preparation:

1. Preheat the oven to 190 ° C. Combine butter, white sugar, and brown sugar in a large bowl until smooth.

2. Beat the egg until everything is well mixed. Mix 1 teaspoon of orange zest and 2 tablespoons of orange juice. Mix the flour, baking powder, and salt; stir in the orange mixture. Mix the cranberries and, if used, the nuts until well distributed. Place the dough per rounded soup spoon on ungreased baking trays.

3. The cookies must be placed at least 2 inches away.

4. Bake in the preheated oven for 12 to 14 minutes, until the edges are golden brown. Remove baking trays to cool on racks. Get a small bowl, mix 1/2 teaspoon of orange peel, 3

tablespoons of orange juice, and icing confectionery ingredients. Spread over cooled cookies. Let's act.

Key Pie Vill

Prep Time: 15 min

Serve: 8

Ingredients:

- 1 (9 inches) prepared graham cracker crust
- 3 cups of sweetened condensed milk
- 1/2 cup sour cream
- 3/4 cup lime juice
- 1 tablespoon grated lime zest

Preparation:

1. Preheat the oven to 175 ° C (350 ° F).

2. Combine the condensed milk, sour cream, lime juice, and lime zest in a medium bowl. Mix well and pour into the graham cracker crust.

3. Bake in the preheated oven for 5 to 8 minutes until small hole bubbles burst on the surface of the cake. DON'T BROWN! Cool the cake well before serving. Decorate with lime slices and whipped cream if desired.

Sweet Popcorn

Prep Time: 5 min

Cook Time: 15 min

Serve: 8

Ingredients:

- 8 cups air-popped popcorn

- 2 tablespoons extra-virgin olive oil

- 2 tablespoons packed brown sugar

- 2 tablespoons Chinese five-spice powder

- 1/4 teaspoon sea salt

Preparation:

1. Preheat the oven to 350°F. Put the popcorn in a large bowl. Set aside. In a small bowl whisk the olive oil brown sugar five-spice powder and sea salt. Pour the mixture over

the popcorn tossing to coat. Transfer to a 9-by- 13-inch baking dish.

2. Bake the popcorn for 15 minutes stirring every 5 minutes or so. Serve hot or cool and store in resealable bags in single-serve (1-cup) batches.

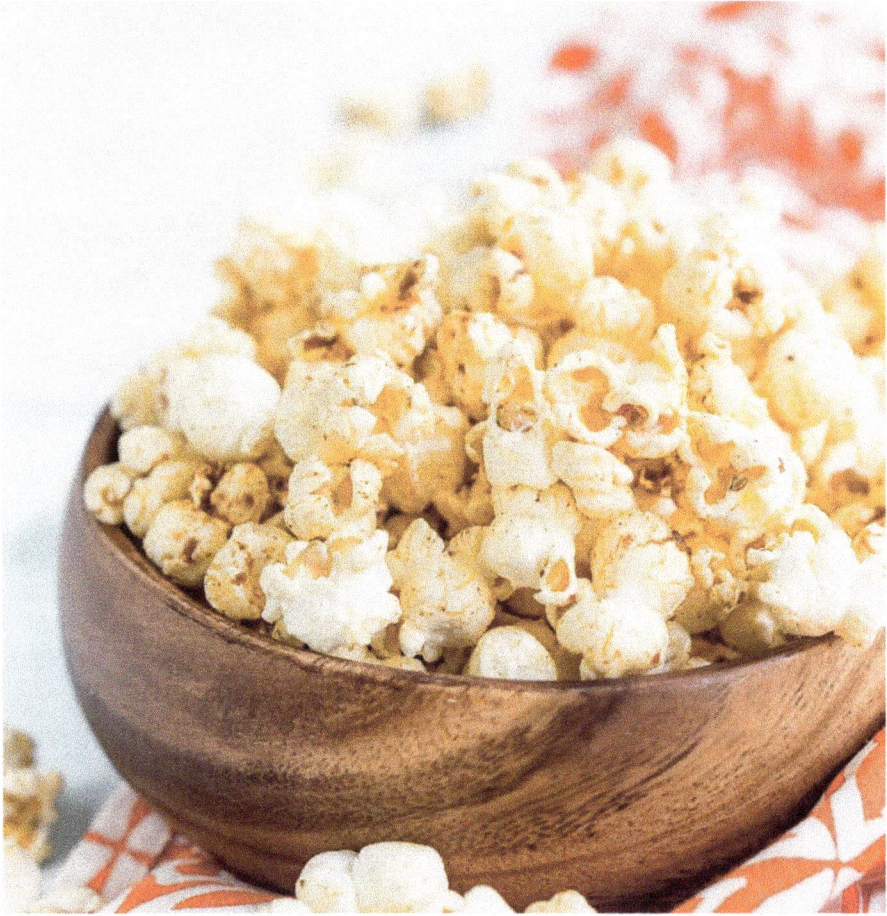

Marinated Olives with Garlic and Thyme

Prep cook Time: 10 min (plus 2 h to marinate)

Serve: 8

Ingredients:

- 1/4 cup extra-virgin olive oil

- 1/4 cup red wine vinegar

- 3 garlic cloves. minced

- 2 tablespoons chopped fresh rosemary leaves

- 1 tablespoon chopped fresh thyme leaves

- Zest of 1 lemon

- 1/2 teaspoon sea salt

- 2 cups black or green olives drained and rinsed

Preparation:

1. In a small bowl whisk the olive oil. vinegar garlic. rosemary. thyme lemon zest and sea salt.

2. Add the olives to your container and pour the marinade over the top. Seal and refrigerate for at least 2 hours. The olives will keep refrigerated for up to 2 weeks.

Authentic Tzatziki Sauce

Prep/Cook Time: 10 min (plus 1 h to chill)

 Serve: 6

Ingredients:

- 1 cup unsweetened nonfat plain Greek yogurt

- 1 cucumber. peeled and grated

- 1 tablespoon chopped fresh dill

- 1 garlic clove minced

- 1/4 teaspoon sea salt

- 1/8 teaspoon freshly ground black pepper

Preparation:

Vigorously whisk the yogurt cucumber. dill. garlic sea salt
and pepper in a small bowl. Cover well and refrigerate for 1
hour or more before serving.

Healthy and Easy Trail Mix

Prep/Cook Time: 10 min

Serve: 8

Ingredients:

- 1/2 cup unsalted roasted cashews

- 1/2 cup walnut halves

- 1/2 cup toasted hazelnuts

- 1/4 cup dried cranberries

- 1/4 cup dried apricots

Preparation:

Mix all the ingredient in a bowl. Store in 1/4 cup servings in resealable bags for up to six weeks.

Kingly Kalamata Karithopita

Prep Time: 15 min

Cook Time: 40 min

Serve: 16

Ingredients:

For the Karithopita (Walnut Cake with Syrup):

- 1¼-cups whole-wheat flour

- 1-tsp ground cinnamon

- 1-tsp baking powder

- ¾-cup white sugar

- ½-tsp salt

- ¼-tsp ground cloves

- ⅓ -cup extra-virgin olive oil (as shortening)

- ¾-cup milk

- 1-pc egg, whisked

- 1-cup walnuts, finely chopped

For the Honey-Lemon Syrup:

- ¼-cup white sugar

- ¼-cup water

- 1-tsp lemon juice

- ¼-cup honey

Preparation:

1. Preheat your oven to 350 °F. Prepare a greased 9" x 9" baking pan. Set aside. Combine and mix the first six Karithopita ingredients in a medium-sized mixing bowl. Mix well until fully incorporated. Transfer the mixture in the mixing bowl of your stand mixer.

2. Pour in the oil, milk, and the egg. Beat the mixture on low speed for 1 minute to a creamy and thick consistency, scraping the mixing bowl's bottom once to avoid lumps.

3. Stir in the chopped walnuts manually using a spatula. Transfer the batter in the prepared baking pan and spread

evenly. Place the pan in the preheated oven. Bake for 40 minutes until an inserted toothpick into the center of the walnut cake comes out clean.

4. Let the walnut cake in the pan cool for 30 minutes. In the meantime, prepare the honey lemon syrup.

For the Lemon Honey-Syrup:

1. Stir in the white sugar with water in a saucepan placed over medium heat. Bring the mixture to a boil. Reduce the heat to low, and allow simmering for 5 minutes.

2. Stir in the lemon juice and honey. Remove the saucepan from the heat. By using a knife, make small slashes in a diamond pattern on the top of the cake. Pour the hot syrup over the walnut cake.

Apple Applied Cinnamon Cake Cooked with Olive Oil

Prep Time: 20 min

Cook Time: 60 min

Serve: 12

Ingredients:

- 4-eggs

- 1-cup brown sugar +2-tbsp for apples

- cup extra-virgin olive oil (as shortening)

- 1-cup milk

- tsp baking powder

- 2½-cups whole-wheat flour

- 1-tsp vanilla extract

- 4-pcs apples, peeled, cored, halved, and sliced thinly

- 1½-tsp ground cinnamon

- ½-cup walnuts, chopped

- ½-cup raisins

- tbsp sesame seeds

Preparation:

1. Preheat your oven to 375 °F. Prepare a greased 9" x 9" baking pan. Set aside. By using your electric hand mixer, beat the eggs and a cup of sugar for 10 minutes. Pour in the olive oil and beat the mixture for 3 minutes.

2. Pour in the milk, and add the baking powder, wheat flour, and vanilla. Beat the mixture for another 3 minutes.

3. Transfer half of the batter in the prepared baking pan and spread evenly. Combine and mix the apples, cinnamon, walnuts, raisins, and the 2-tbsp of brown sugar in a mixing bowl. Mix thoroughly until fully combined.

4. Transfer the apple mixture over the batter in the baking pan and spread evenly. Top the apple mixture with the

remaining batter. Sprinkle the batter with the sesame seeds.

5. Place the pan in the preheated oven. Bake for 50 minutes until an inserted toothpick into the center of the apple-cinnamon cake comes out clean.

Naturally Nutty & Buttery

Banana Bowl

Prep Time: 5 min

Cook Time: 0 min

Serve: 4

Ingredients:

- 4- cups vanilla Greek yogurt

- 2-pcs medium-sized bananas, sliced

- ¼-cup creamy and natural peanut butter

- 1-tsp ground nutmeg

- ¼-cup flaxseed meal

Preparation:

1. Divide the yogurt equally between four serving bowls. Top each yogurt bowl with the banana slices.

2. Place the peanut butter in a microwave-safe bowl. Melt the peanut butter in your microwave for 40 seconds. Drizzle one tablespoon of the melted peanut butter over the bananas for each bowl. To serve, sprinkle over with the ground nutmeg and flax-seed meal.

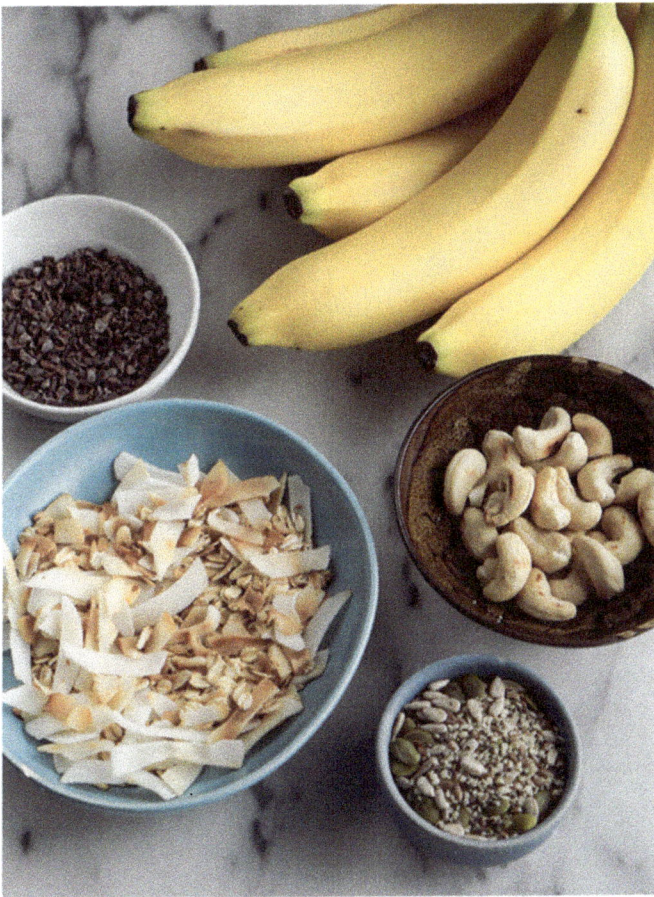

Queenly Quinoa Choco Crunch Baked Bars

Prep Time: 5 min

Cook Time: 20 min

Servings: 10

Ingredients:

- 2½-tbsp peanut butter with roasted peanuts

- 2-tbsp water

- 1-lb. semi-sweet chocolate bars, chopped into small pieces

- 1-cup dry quinoa

- ½-tsp vanilla

- 1-tbsp natural peanut butter

Preparation:

1. Preheat for 10 minutes a heavy-bottomed pot placed over medium-high heat. Meanwhile, prepare a baking sheet lined with parchment paper. Set aside.

2. Make a peanut butter drizzle by stirring the peanut butter with roasted peanuts with water in a small mixing bowl until fully incorporated. Set aside.

3. Add the quinoa by batch, ¼-cup at a time to pop. Allow each batch to sit at the bottom of the pot, stirring occasionally. Once the quinoa starts to pop, swirl it constantly for 1 minute until the popping subsides. (This can happen too quickly, so ensure to take it off lest the quinoa turns brown.) Set aside.

4. Place the chopped chocolate bars in a microwave-safe mixing bowl. Melt it in your microwave for 30 seconds.

5. Add the popped quinoa, vanilla, and peanut butter in the mixing bowl of the melted chocolate. Mix thoroughly until fully combined. Transfer the chocolate-quinoa mixture in

the prepared baking sheet. You need not spread the mixture across the sheet; else, it gets too thin. Simply form a roughly square shape of the mixture, about half an inch thick, in the middle of the sheet.

6. Pour the peanut butter drizzle over chocolate-quinoa square. By using a spatula, spread gently the drizzle entirely around the square.

7. Refrigerate the mixture for an hour until it becomes completely a firm cake. To serve, slice the cake into small square bars.

Phyllo Pastry Balkan Baklava

Prep Time: 30 min

Cook Time: 35 min

Serve: 18

Ingredients:

For the Baklava:

- 12-sheets phyllo pastry dough

- 1-tsp ground cloves

- 2-tsp ground cinnamon

- 2-cups walnuts, chopped

- 1-cup sesame seeds

- 2-cups almonds, chopped

- 3-tbsp honey

- 1-cup extra-virgin olive oil (for brushing the dough)

- 18-pcs whole cloves (1 for each piece of baklava slice)

For the Honey Syrup:

- 1-pc lemon, rind

- 1-cinnamon stick

- 2-cups sugar

- 1-cup honey

- 2-cups water

- 2- pc lemon, juice

Preparation:

For the Baklava:

1. Preheat your oven to 350 °F. Mix the ground cloves, cinnamon, walnuts, sesame seeds and almonds with honey in a mixing bowl. Brush with olive oil 4-sheets of phyllo pastry, on both sides of each. Lay the oiled sheets on top of each other in a 9" x 9" baking pan.

2. Transfer half of the nut mixture on top of the oiled sheets and spread evenly. Brush with olive oil another set of 4-

sheets of phyllo pastry, on both sides. Lay this set of oiled sheets over the nut mixture.

3. Empty the mixing bowl with the remaining nut mixture over the oiled sheets and spread evenly. Top the nut mixture with the last set of 4-sheets of phyllo pastry, brushed in the same manner as the other previous sets.

4. Slice the baklava into 18-equally sized pieces. Top each slice with one whole clove.

5. Place the baking pan in the preheated oven. Bake for 35 minutes until the top turns golden brown. Prepare for the honey syrup while the baklava is baking.

For the Honey Syrup:

1. Combine the lemon peel, cinnamon stick, and sugar with honey and water in a saucepan placed over medium heat.

2. Bring the mixture to a boil. Reduce the heat to low, and simmer for 15 minutes. Let the syrup to cool down before stirring in the lemon juice.

Baked Apple Delight

Prep Time: 10 min

Cook Time: 1 h

Serve: 6

Ingredients:

- 6 Apples

- 3 Tablespoons Almonds, Chopped

- 1/3 Cup Cherries, Dried & Chopped Coarsely

- 1 Tablespoon Wheat Germ

- 1 Tablespoon Brown Sugar

- ¼ Cup Water

- ½ Cup Apple Juice

- 1/8 Teaspoon Nutmeg

- ½ Teaspoon Cinnamon

- 2 Tablespoons Dark Honey, Raw

- 2 Teaspoons Walnut Oil

Preparation:

1. Start by heating your oven to 350, and then blend your almonds, wheat germ, brown sugar, cherries, nutmeg and cinnamon in a bowl. Set this bowl to the side.

2. Core your apples starting from their stem, and chop into ¾ inch pieces. Place this mixture into each hole.

3. Arrange the apples upright in a baking dish. A small one will work best. Pour in your apple juice and water, and then drizzle the oil and honey over top.

4. Cover with foil, and cook for fifty to sixty minutes. The apples should be tender. Serve at room temperature or immediately.

Crepes with passion fruit

Prep Time: 5 min

Cook Time: 10 min

Serve: 4

Ingredients:

- Crepes

- Sauce

- Two eggs

- 1/25 cups oat milk

- 1 cup flour

- 1/5 tbsp butter

- ½ cup of sugar

- ¾ cup of passion fruit

Preparation:

1. Mix eggs, milk, and flour and keep it aside. Mix sugar with passion fruit and boil it to reduce the concentration to half.

2. Melt the butter and spread crepe mixture in a pan and cook for 2 minutes from both sides.

3. Transfer the crepe to a plate with sauce and serve.

Fennel and seared scallop's salad

Prep Time: 30 min

Cook Time: 10 min

Serve: 4

Ingredients:

- One grapefruit

- 1 tbsp olive oil

- 1 tsp raw honey

- 1/2 tsp chopped fennel seeds

- 1/4 tsp sea salt

- Pinch of black pepper

- 12 sea scallops

- 1/2 sliced

- 3 cups torn red leaf lettuce

- 12 toasted almonds

Preparation:

1. Strain the grapefruit juice in a cup. For the dressing: Transfer juice into a small bowl & whisk oil, add water, honey, fennel, salt & black pepper.

2. Set it aside. Season scallops with remaining fennel & remaining salt.

3. Heat skillet & brush with remaining oil. Cook scallops for five minutes, flipping halfway, till they become lightly from both sides. Transfer it to a plate & cover it. Repeat the same with remaining. Set aside the dressing. In a bowl, toss the fennel & lettuce with the remaining dressing. Divide the fennel salad among the serving plates. Top each salad with the grapefruit pieces & cooked scallops.

4. Drizzle the reserved dressing over scallops & top with the almonds.

Fruity asparagus quinoa salad

Prep Time: 15 min

Cook Time: 5 min

Serve: 7

Ingredients:

- 2 cups cooked quinoa

- 3 tsp olive oil

- 30 sliced spears asparagus

- 1/2 tsp salt

- 1/4 tsp pepper

- Two cloves garlic

- Salt and pepper

- 16 sliced strawberries

- 4.5 oz mozzarella cheese

- 1/3 cup Balsamic Vinaigrette

- 2 tbsp basil

Preparation:

1. Place cooked quinoa in a bowl. Prepare the balsamic vinaigrette & set aside. Heat olive oil in a pan to overheat.

2. Once heated, add asparagus & garlic. Sprinkle with salt & pepper. Cook 2-3 min. Add asparagus to quinoa.

3. Mix the strawberries, balsamic vinaigrette & cheese.

4. Toss to mix well. Top salad with the basil.

Curried Veggies and Poached Eggs

Prep Time: 20 min

Cook Time: 45 min

Serve: 4

Ingredients:

- 4 large eggs

- ½ tsp. white vinegar

- 1/8 tsp. crushed red pepper – optional

- 1 cup water

- 1 14-oz. can chickpeas, drained

- 2 medium zucchinis, diced

- ½ lb. sliced button mushrooms

- 1 tbsp. yellow curry powder

- 2 cloves garlic, minced

- 1 large onion, chopped

- 2 tsp.s. extra virgin olive oil

Preparation:

1. On medium high fire, place a large saucepan and heat oil. Sauté onions until tender around four to five minutes.

2. Add garlic and continue sautéing for another half minute.

3. Add curry powder, stir and cook until fragrant around one to two minutes. Add mushrooms, mix, cover and cook for 5 to 8 minutes or until mushrooms are tender and have released their liquid.

4. Add red pepper if using, water, chickpeas and zucchini.

5. Mix well to combine and bring to a boil.

Once boiling, reduce fire to a simmer, cover and cook until zucchini is tender around 15 to 20 minutes of simmering.

6. Meanwhile, in a small pot filled with 3-inches deep water, bring to a boil on high fire. Once boiling, reduce fire to a simmer and add vinegar.

7. Slowly add one egg, slipping it gently into the water. Allow to simmer until egg is cooked, around 3 to 5 minutes.

8. Remove egg with a slotted spoon and transfer to a plate, one plate one egg. Repeat the process with remaining eggs.

9. Once the veggies are done cooking, divide evenly into 4 servings and place one serving per egg plate. Serve and enjoy.

Eggs over Kale Hash

Prep Time: 10 min

Cook Time: 20 min

Serve: 4

Ingredients:

- 4 large eggs

- 1 bunch chopped kale

- Dash of ground nutmeg

- 2 sweet potatoes, cubed

- 1 14.5-ounce can of chicken broth

Preparation:

1. In a large non-stick skillet, bring the chicken broth to a simmer. Add the sweet potatoes and season slightly with salt and pepper.

2. Add a dash of nutmeg to improve the flavor. Cook until the sweet potatoes become soft, around 10 minutes. Add kale and season with salt and pepper. Continue cooking for four minutes or until kale has wilted. Set aside.

3. Using the same skillet, heat 1 tablespoon of olive oil over medium high heat. Cook the eggs sunny side up until the whites become opaque and the yolks have set. Top the kale hash with the eggs. Serve immediately.

Italian Scrambled Eggs

Prep Time: 10 min

Cook Time: 7 min

Serve: 1

Ingredients:

- 1 teaspoon balsamic vinegar

- 2 large eggs

- ¼ teaspoon rosemary, minced

- ½ cup cherry tomatoes

- 1 ½ cup kale, chopped

- ½ teaspoon olive oil

Preparation:

1. Melt the olive oil in a skillet over medium high heat.

2. Sauté the kale and add rosemary and salt to taste. Add three tablespoons of water to prevent the kale from burning at the bottom of the pan. Cook for three to four minutes.

3. Add the tomatoes and stir.

4. Push the vegetables on one side of the skillet and add the eggs. Season with salt and pepper to taste.

5. Scramble the eggs then fold in the tomatoes and kales.

Lettuce Stuffed with Eggs 'n Crab Meat

Prep Time: 15 min

Cook Time: 10 min

Serve: 8

Ingredients:

- 24 butter lettuce leaves

- 1 tsp. dry mustard

- ¼ cup finely chopped celery

- 1 cup lump crabmeat, around 5 ounces

- 3 tbsp. plain Greek yogurt

- 2 tbsp. extra virgin olive oil

- ¼ tsp. ground pepper

- 8 large eggs

- ½ tsp. salt, divided

- 1 tbsp. fresh lemon juice, divided

- 2 cups thinly sliced radishes

Preparation:

1. In a medium bowl, mix ¼ tsp. salt, 2 tsp.s. Juice and radishes. Cover and chill for half an hour.

2. On medium saucepan, place eggs and cover with water over an inch above the eggs. Bring the pan of water to a boil. Once boiling, reduce fire to a simmer and cook for ten minutes. Turn off fire, discard hot water and place eggs in an ice water bath to cool completely.

3. Peel eggshells and slice eggs in half lengthwise and remove the yolks. With a sieve on top of a bowl, place yolks and press through a sieve. Set aside a tablespoon of yolk.

4. On remaining bowl of yolks add pepper, ¼ tsp. salt and 1 tsp. juice. Mix well and as you are stirring, slowly add oil until well incorporated. Add yogurt, stir well to mix.

5. Add mustard, celery and crabmeat. Gently mix to combine. If needed, taste and adjust seasoning of the filling.

6. On a serving platter, arrange 3 lettuces in a fan for two egg slices. To make the egg whites sit flat, you can slice a bit of the bottom to make it flat. Evenly divide crab filling into egg white holes.

7. Then evenly divide into eight servings the radish salad and add on the eggs' side, on top of the lettuce leaves.

Serve and enjoy.

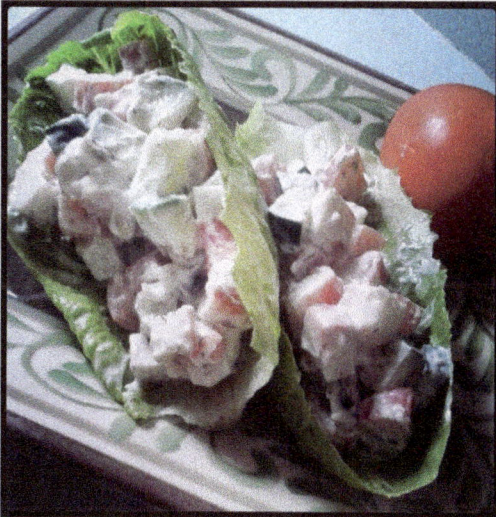

Parmesan and Poached Eggs

on Asparagus

Prep Time: 10 min

Cook Time: 15 min

Serve: 4

Ingredients:

- 4 tbsp. coarsely grated fresh

- Parmesan cheese, divided

- Freshly ground black pepper, to taste

- 2 tsp.s. finely chopped fresh parsley

- 2 tbsp. fresh lemon juice

- 1 tbsp. unsalted butter

- 1 garlic clove, chopped

- 1 tbsp. extra virgin olive oil

- 2 bunches asparagus spears, trimmed around 40

- 1 tsp. salt, divided

- 1 tsp. white vinegar

- 8 large eggs

Preparation:

1. Break eggs and place in one paper cup per egg. On medium high fire, place a low sided pan filled 3/4 with water. Add ½ tsp. salt and vinegar into water. Set aside.

2. On medium high fire bring another pot of water to boil.

3. Once boiling, lower fire to a simmer and blanch asparagus until tender and crisp, around 3-4 minutes. With tongs transfer asparagus to a serving platter and set aside.

4. On medium fire, place a medium saucepan and heat olive oil. Once hot, for a minute sauté garlic and turn off fire. Add butter right away and swirl around pan to melt. Add remaining pepper, salt, parsley and lemon juice and mix thoroughly. Add asparagus and toss to combine well

with garlic butter sauce. Transfer to serving platter along with sauce.

5. In boiling pan of water, poach the eggs by pouring eggs into the water slowly and cook for two minutes per egg.

6. With a slotted spoon, remove egg, remove excess water, tap slotted spoon several times on kitchen towel, and place it on top of asparagus.

7. To serve, top eggs with parmesan cheese and divide the asparagus into two and 2 eggs per plate. Serve and enjoy.

Scrambled eggs with Smoked Salmon

Prep Time: 15 min

Cook Time: 8 min

Serve: 1

Ingredients:

- 1 tbsp. coconut oil

- Pepper and salt to taste

- 1/8 tsp. red pepper flakes

- 1/8 tsp. garlic powder

- 1 tbsp. fresh dill, chopped finely

- 4 oz. smoked salmon, torn apart

- 2 whole eggs + 1 egg yolk, whisked

Preparation:

1. In a big bowl whisk the eggs. Mix in pepper, salt, red pepper flakes, garlic, dill and salmon.

2. On low fire, place a nonstick fry pan and lightly grease with oil. Pour egg mixture and whisk around until cooked through to make scrambled eggs, around 8 minutes on medium fire. Serve and enjoy.

Scrambled Eggs with Feta 'n Mushrooms

Prep Time: 5 min

Cook Time: 6 min

Serve: 1

Ingredients:

- Pepper to taste

- 2 tbsp. feta cheese

- 1 whole egg

- 2 egg whites

- 1 cup fresh spinach, chopped

- ½ cup fresh mushrooms, sliced

- Cooking spray

Preparation:

1. On medium high fire, place a nonstick fry pan and grease with cooking spray. Once hot, add spinach and mushrooms.

2. Sauté until spinach is wilted, around 2-3 minutes.

3. Meanwhile, in a bowl whisk well egg, egg whites, and cheese. Season with pepper.

4. Pour egg mixture into pan and scramble until eggs are cooked through, around 3-4 minutes.

5. Serve and enjoy with a piece of toast or brown rice.

Belly-Filling Cajun Rice & Chicken

Prep Time: 15 min

Cook Time: 20 min

Serve: 6

Ingredients:

- 1 tablespoon oil

- 1 onion, diced

- 3 cloves of garlic, minced

- 1-pound chicken breasts, sliced

- 1 tablespoon Cajun seasoning

- 1 tablespoon tomato paste

- 2 cups chicken broth

- 1 ½ cups white rice, rinsed

- 1 bell pepper, chopped

Preparation:

1. Press the Sauté on the Instant Pot and pour the oil. Sauté the onion and garlic until fragrant.

2. Stir in the chicken breasts and season with Cajun seasoning. Continue cooking for 3 minutes. Add the tomato paste and chicken broth. Dissolve the tomato paste before adding the rice and bell pepper.

3. Close the lid and press the rice button. Once done cooking, do a natural release for 10 minutes. Then, do a quick release.

4. Once cooled, evenly divide into serving size, keep in your preferred container, and refrigerate until ready to eat.

The Bell Pepper Fiesta

Prep Time: 10 min

Cook Time: 0 min

Serve: 4

Ingredients:

tablespoons dill, chopped

- 1 yellow onion, chopped
- 1 pound multi colored peppers, cut, halved, seeded and cut into thin strips
- tablespoons organic olive oil
- ½ tablespoons white wine vinegar
- Black pepper to taste

Preparation:

Take a bowl and mix in sweet pepper, onion, dill, pepper, oil, vinegar and toss well. Divide between bowls and serve.

Dal with Kale, Red Onions and Buckwheat

Prep Time: 5 min

Cook Time: 20 min

Serve: 2

Ingredients:

- 1 teaspoon of extra virgin olive oil

- 1 teaspoon of mustard seeds

- 40g red onions, finely chopped

- 1 clove of garlic, very finely chopped

- 1 teaspoon very finely chopped ginger

- 1 Thai chili, very finely chopped

- 1 teaspoon curry mixture teaspoons turmeric

- 300ml vegetable broth

- 40g red lentils

- 50g kale, chopped

- 50ml coconut milk

- 50g buckwheat

Preparation:

1. Heat oil in a pan Add the curry powder and 1 teaspoon of turmeric, mix well.

2. Add the vegetable stock, bring to the boil.

3. Add the lentils and cook them for 25 to 30 minutes until they are ready. Then add the kale and coconut milk and simmer for 5 minutes. The Dal is ready.

Spiced Up Pumpkin Seeds Bowls

Prep Time: 10 min

Cook Time: 20 min

Serve: 4

Ingredients:

- ½ tablespoon chili powder
- ½ teaspoon cayenne
- cups pumpkin seeds
- teaspoons lime juice

Preparation:

1. Spread pumpkin seeds over lined baking sheet; add lime juice, cayenne and chili powder. Toss well.

2. Pre-heat your oven to 275 degrees F. Roast in your oven for 20 minutes and transfer to small bowls.

3. Serve and enjoy!

Chicken & Bean Casserole

Prep Time: 5 min

Cook Time: 40 min

Serve: 2

Ingredients:

- 400g 14oz chopped tomatoes
- 400g 14 oz. tinned cannellini beans or haricot beans
- chicken thighs, skin removed
- carrots, peeled and finely chopped
- red onions, chopped
- sticks of celery large mushrooms
- red peppers bell peppers, deseeded and chopped
- 1 clove of garlic
- tablespoons soy sauce
- 1 tablespoon olive oil

- liters 3 pints chicken stock broth

Preparation:

1. Heat the olive oil. Add the garlic and onions and cook for 5 minutes. Add in the chicken, carrots, cannellini beans, celery, red peppers bell peppers and mushrooms.

2. Pour in the stock broth soy sauce and tomatoes.

3. Bring it to the boil. Serve.

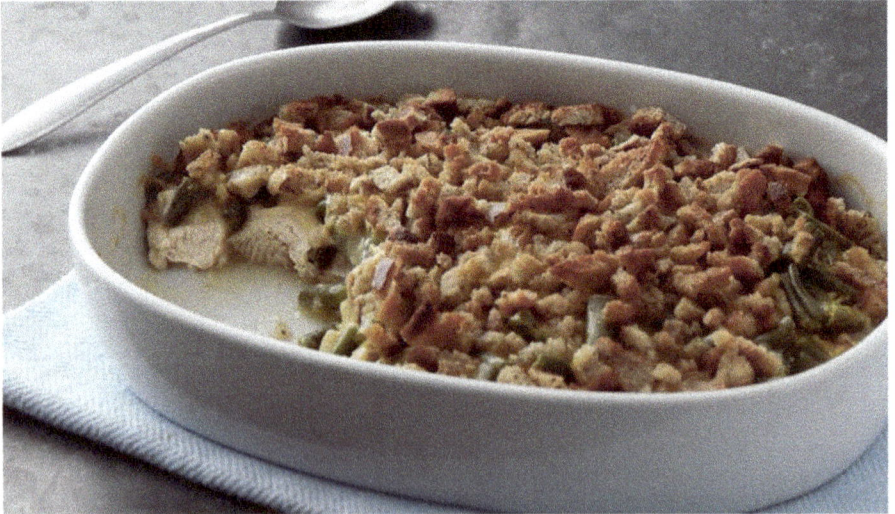

Chicken Salad

Prep Time: 5 min

Cook Time: 30 min

Serve: 2

Ingredients:

- ½ red onion, very finely sliced

- 1 tablespoon of sesame seeds

- 150g of cooked chicken-shredded Large handful

- 20g of parsley-chopped

- 100g of baby kale-chopped roughly

- teaspoons of soy sauce

- 1 teaspoon of clear honey

- 1 teaspoon of sesame oil

Preparation:

1. Place a frying pan over medium heat. Mix the sesame oil, honey, olive oil, lime juice, and soy sauce to make the dressing. Place the cucumber, red onion, kale, pak choi, and parsley in a large bowl and gently mix.

2. Pour the dressing over and mix again.

Tuna, Egg & Caper Salad

Prep Time: 5 min

Cook Time: 20 min

Serve: 2

Ingredients:

- 100g 3½oz. red chicory or yellow if not available

- 150g 5oz tinned tuna flakes in brine, drained

- 100g 3 ½ oz. cucumber

- 25g 1oz rocket arugula pitted black olives

- hard-boiled eggs, peeled and quartered

- tomatoes, chopped

- tablespoons fresh parsley, chopped

- 1 red onion, chopped

- 1 stalk of celery

- 1 tablespoon capers

- tablespoons garlic vinaigrette see recipe

- 340 calories per serving

Preparation:

1. Place the tuna, cucumber, olives, tomatoes, onion, chicory, celery, parsley, and rocket arugula into a bowl.

2. Serve onto plates and scatter the eggs and capers on top.

Mussels in Red Wine Sauce

Prep Time: 5 min

Cook Time: 50 min

Serve: 2

Ingredients:

- 800g 2lb mussels

- x 400g 14 oz. tins of chopped tomatoes

- 25g 1oz butter

- 1 tablespoon fresh chives, chopped

- 1 tablespoon fresh parsley, chopped

- 1 bird's-eye chili, finely chopped

- cloves of garlic, crushed

- 400 ml 14fl. oz. red wine

- Juice of 1 lemon

Preparation:

1. Heat the butter in a large saucepan and add in the red wine. Reduce the heat and add the parsley, chives, chili and garlic while stirring.

2. Add in the tomatoes, lemon juice and mussels. Cover the saucepan and cook for 2-3 minutes. Serve.

Roast Balsamic Vegetables

Prep Time: 5 min

Cook Time: 45 min

Serve: 2

Ingredients:

- tomatoes, chopped

- red onions, chopped

- sweet potatoes, peeled and chopped

- 100g 3½ oz. red chicory or if unavailable, use yellow

- 100g 3½ oz. kale, finely chopped

- 300g 11oz potatoes, peeled and chopped

- stalks of celery, chopped

- 1 bird's-eye chili, de-seeded and finely chopped

- tablespoons fresh parsley, chopped

- tablespoons fresh coriander cilantro chopped

- tablespoons olive oil

- tablespoons balsamic vinegar

- 1 teaspoon mustard

- Sea salt

- Freshly ground black pepper

Preparation:

1. Place the olive oil, balsamic, mustard, parsley and coriander cilantro into a bowl and mix well.

2. Toss all the remaining ingredients into the dressing and season with salt and pepper. Serve.

Salmon and Capers

Prep Time: 10 min

Cook Time: 0

Serve: 4

Ingredients:

- 75g (3oz) Greek yogurt

- salmon fillets, skin removed

- teaspoons Dijon Mustard

- 1 tablespoon capers, chopped

- teaspoons fresh parsley

- Zest of 1 lemon

Preparation:

1. In a bowl, mix the yogurt, mustard, lemon zest, parsley and capers. Thoroughly coat the salmon in the mixture.

2. Place the salmon under a hot grill (broiler) and cook for 3-4 minutes on each side, or until the fish is cooked.

3. Serve with mashed potatoes and vegetables or a large green leafy salad.

Rocket salad with Tuna

Prep Time: 5 min

Cook Time: 15 min

Serve: 4

Ingredients:

- slices rustic bread, torn into pieces

- large tomatoes

- Tbsp. olive oil

- 400g tin cannellini beans, drained and rinsed

- ¼ cup Kalamata olives

- cups shredded rocket

- ¼ red onion, sliced finely

- 85g tin tuna

Dressing:

- Tbsp. olive oil

- ½ tsp. dijon mustard

- 1 Tbsp. lemon juice

Preparation:

1. Start with setting the oven at 180C.

2. Place the bread slices in braking tray, put olive oil on slices and bake for 10-15 mins.

3. To prepare the dressing mix lemon juice, mustard and oil in a jar. Bring a bowl, add baked bread, onions, beans, tuna, tomatoes and rocket. Put the dressing over salad and enjoy.

Sirt Super Salad

Prep Time: 5 min

Cook Time: 15 min

Serve: 1

Ingredients:

- 1 3⁄4 ounces (50g) arugula

- 1⁄2 ounces (100g) smoked salmon slices

- 1 3⁄4 ounces (50g) endive leaves

- 1⁄2 cup (50g) celery including leaves, sliced

- 1⁄8 cups (15g) walnuts, chopped

- 1⁄2 cup (80g) avocado, peeled, stoned, and sliced

- 1⁄8 cup (20g) red onion, sliced

- 1 tablespoon extra-virgin olive oil

- 1 tablespoon capers

- 1 large Medjool date, pitted and chopped

- 1⁄4 cup (10g) parsley, chopped

- Juice of 1⁄4 lemon

Preparation:

Bring a bowl, place large leaves of salad, add all the ingredients one by one in the bowl and stir through the bowl and enjoy.

Strawberry Buckwheat Tabbouleh

Prep Time: 5 min

Cook Time: 15 min

Serve: 1

Ingredients:

- ⅓ cup (50g) buckwheat

- ½ cup (80g) avocado

- 1 tablespoon ground turmeric

- ⅛ cup (20g) red onion

- ⅜ cup (65g) tomato

- 1 tablespoon capers

- ⅛ cup (25g) Medjool dates, pitted

- ⅔ cup (100g) strawberries, hulled

- ¾ cup (30g) parsley

- 1 tablespoon extra-virgin olive oil

- 1 ounce (30g) arugula

- Juice of ½ lemon

Preparation:

1. Start with cooking the buckwheat by mixing the turmeric according to the instructions of package. Drain and let it cool. Now, start chopping the tomatoes, capers, onions, avocados, dates and parsley. Mix all of them with already cooked buckwheat.

2. After that, take the strawberries, slice them and add them in salad. Garnish the salad on the arugula bed.

Fragrant Anise Hotpot Sirtfood

Prep Time: 2 min

Cook Time: 10 min

Serve: 2

Ingredients:

- 1 tbsp. tomato purée

- 1 star anise, crushed (or 1/4 tsp ground anise)

- Small handful (10g) parsley, stalks finely chopped

- Small handful (10g) coriander, stalks finely chopped

- Juice of 1/2 lime

- 1/2 carrot, peeled and cut into matchsticks

- 500ml chicken stock, fresh or made with

- 1 cube 50g beansprouts

- 100g firm tofu, chopped

- 50g broccoli, cut into small florets

- 100g raw tiger prawns

- 50g cooked water chestnuts, drained

- 50g rice noodles, cooked according to packet instructions

- 1 tbsp. good-quality miso paste

- 20g sushi ginger, chopped

Preparation:

1. Take a pan and put the parsley stalks, lime juice, tomato purée, coriander stalks, star anise, and chicken stock, let them simmer for 10-12 mins.

2. Now add the broccoli, tofu, carrot, water, chestnuts, and prawns, gently mix them and let them cook completely.

3. Turn off the heat and add in the miso paste and sushi ginger. Garnish with coriander and parsley leaves.

Coronation Chicken Salad

Prep Time: 2 min

Cook Time: 2 min

Serve: 1

Ingredients:

- 75 g Natural yoghurt

- 1 tsp. Coriander, chopped

- Juice of 1/4 of a lemon

- 1/2 tsp. Mild curry powder

- 1 tsp. Ground turmeric

- Walnut halves, finely chopped

- 100 g Cooked chicken breast, cut into bite-sized pieces

- 20 g Red onion, diced

- 1 Bird's eye chili

- 1 Medjool date, finely chopped

- 40 g Rocket, to serve

Preparation:

Take a bowl, gather the ingredients, mix them in bowl, and serve the salad on the rocket bedding.

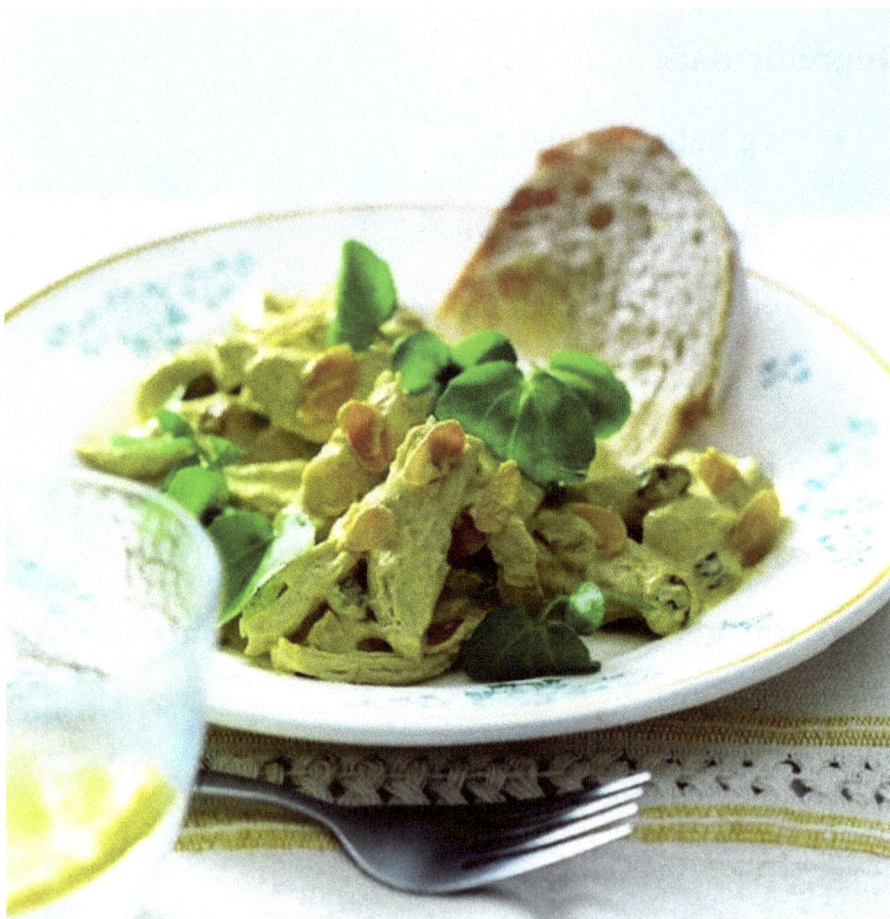

Buckwheat Pasta Salad

Prep Time: 15 min

Cook Time: 0 min

Serve: 1

Ingredients:

- 50g cooked buckwheat pasta

- small handful of basil leaves

- large handful of rockets

- 1/2 avocado, diced

- 1 tbsp. extra virgin olive oil

- 20g pine nuts

- cherry tomatoes, halved olives

Preparation:

Take a bowl or a plate, add in all the ingredients, now scatter the pine nuts all over the ingredients and serve.

Shrimp Pasta

Prep Time: 45 min

Cook Time: 10 min

Serve: 2

Ingredients:

- ounces linguine

- ¼ cup mayonnaise

- ¼ cup bean stew glue

- Two cloves garlic, squashes

- ½ pound shrimp, stripped

- One teaspoon salt

- ½ teaspoon cayenne pepper

- One teaspoon garlic powder

- One tablespoon vegetable oil

- One lime, squeezed

- ¼ cup green onion, slashed

- ¼ cup cilantro, minced

- Red bean stew chips, for embellish

Preparation:

1. Cook pasta still somewhat firm as per box guidelines. In a little bowl, consolidate mayonnaise, stew glue and garlic. Race to join. Put in a safe spot. In a blending bowl, include shrimp, salt, cayenne and garlic powder.

2. Mix to cover shrimp. Oil in a heavy skillet over medium warmth. Include shrimp and cook for around 2 minutes to flip and cook for an extra 2 minutes. Add pasta and sauce to the dish. Mood killer the warmth and combine until the pasta is covered.

Chicken Thighs with Creamy Tomato Spinach Sauce

Prep Time: 45 min

Cook Time: 10 min

Serve: 2

Ingredients:

- One tablespoon olive oil
- lb. chicken thighs, boneless skinless
- ½ teaspoon salt
- ¼ teaspoon pepper
- oz. tomato sauce
- Two garlic cloves, minced
- ½ cup overwhelming cream
- oz. new spinach

- Four leaves fresh basil (or utilize ¼ teaspoon dried basil)

Preparation:

1. The most effective method to cook boneless skinless chicken thighs in a skillet: In a much skillet heat olive oil on medium warmth. Boneless chicken with salt and pepper. Add top side down to the hot skillet.

2. Cook for 5 minutes on medium heat, until the high side, is pleasantly burned. Flip over to the opposite side and heat for five additional minutes on medium heat. Expel the chicken from the skillet to a plate.

3. Step by step instructions to make creamy tomato basil sauce: To the equivalent, presently void skillet, include tomato sauce, minced garlic, and substantial cream. Bring to bubble and mix. Lessen warmth to low stew. Include new spinach and new basil. Mix until spinach withers and diminishes in volume. Taste the sauce and include

progressively salt and pepper, if necessary. Include back cooked boneless skinless chicken thighs, increment warmth to medium.